D0067978

THE PALEO KID LUNCH BOX:

27 Kid-Approved Recipes That Make Lunchtime A Breeze

(Primal Gluten Free Kids Cookbook)

Kate Evans Scott

KIDS LOVE PRESS

Copyright © 2013 Kids Love Press
All Rights Reserved.
ISBN-13: 978-0-9919729-2-0

This book is dedicated to my two beautiful children.

TABLE OF CONTENTS

MAKE-AHEAD RECIPES

QUICK-PACK RECIPES

BEVERAGES

ACKNOWLEDGMENTS

Thanks to everyone who helped make this book a reality. My gratitude also goes out to those living the Paleo lifestyle - your support has been the cornerstone of this creative process.

THE PALEO LUNCH BOX

Often you will hear that breakfast is the most important meal of the day, but for children who wake up early and go off to school, lunch can be just as vital.

Kids Need A Healthy Lunch

By the time the lunch bell rings, that nutritious breakfast has already been used up, and your child will need to eat again to have enough energy for the activities of the afternoon. When children regularly skip lunch or eat lunches devoid of vital nutrients, they become tired and sluggish until they get to their afternoon snack or evening meal. This kind of fatigue often causes learning delays, headaches, irritability, and even obesity.

PREPARING YOUR KIDS FOR LUNCHTIME AT SCHOOL

As a Paleo parent, you likely already understand the importance of a healthy, nutrient-rich diet for your child's physical and cognitive development. But do you also understand the impact of lunchtime on your child's social life?

In a typical school, lunch is one of the few times during the day where children sit together in an unstructured environment, free to chat and laugh and, unfortunately, scrutinize each other's lunches.

"I'll trade you my bologna for your PBJ!"

"I got a chocolate chip cookie! What did you get?"

While schools try to crack down on any lunch sharing, you'll still hear these things around the elementary school cafeteria. First, you'll want to maintain a dialogue with your child about the importance of the healthy lifestyle you've chosen and the negative effects of refined sugars and grains. Ultimately, you won't be able to stay by your child's side all the time, so you want them to be confident in their choice to stick to their Paleo foods.

Second, you'll want to pack lunches that are delicious and exciting so they won't have any reason to trade for a snack cake or a processed meat sandwich. They'll be proud of their lunch, feel full and energized, and look forward to opening the lid of their lunch box every day!

Involvement Fosters Responsibility

For older children and teens, this gets even trickier. They might be tempted by the pizza and French fries sold in the lunch line. They'll also be more likely to skip lunch all together in favor of hanging outside with their friends or engaging in another activity, like wrapping up homework or shooting hoops. Just keep up the conversations, point them to health and nutrition web sites, and most importantly- keep them involved in their own food preparations. They're more likely to eat what they've chosen for themselves.

Give them the recipes for items like spice cookies, fruit leathers, and trail mix granola bars. Have them prepare a batch a week so they have something quick to grab that's going to provide them with some protein and refuel them for the rest of the day, even if they're on the run at lunch time. Remember, when they make it themselves, they are more likely to enjoy it and be proud of their food creation!

PACKING A PALEO LUNCH

Packing a Paleo lunch will take a little bit of planning on your part. You'll want to have a few staples on hand like boiled eggs and lunch meats, as well as lots of fresh fruits and vegetables. Please remember that a Paleo eater will always try to eat grass-fed, free range, organic meats, poultry and eggs. Fruits and vegetables should also be organic, and as local as possible. Here's a list of simple staples that I like to have on hand all the time, for lunches and for snacks:

Simple Staples:

- Boiled eggs
- Peeled, cut vegetables
- Fresh fruits
- Dried fruits
- Nuts and seeds
- Cooked meats

Prepackaged Staples:

While prepackaged foods are generally avoided on a Paleo diet, there are a few that will work in a pinch. If you have a child that seems to be caught up on her friend's colorfully packaged gummy fruits and candy-coated granola bars, occasionally throwing in one of these options might help her feel more like her peers and stay excited about her Paleo lifestyle.

If you are sticking very strictly to the Paleo diet, you will want to stay organic and fresh... but it's my experience that giving a little on this will help keep your child on board long term.

- LARA bars (make sure it's the grain-free variety)
- Applesauce pouches
- Individually packaged nuts (without oils)
- Pure fruit smoothie drinks (no added sugars or artificial ingredients)
- 100% fruit leathers

Packaging:

You'll also need to have a lunch box, bento box, or lunch bags and various containers and packaging to make your lunch packing a snap.

- Bento box
- Lunch box
- Reusable freezer packs
- Wax paper
- Cello or plastic bags
- Parchment paper
- Thermos
- Utensils
- Insulated water bottle

My favorite lunch box is a thermal type that holds a bento box inside. You can use it with or without the bento box, and it keeps perishable items cold. Because the box lays down flat instead of standing on its side like a traditional lunch box, you can comfortably eat right out of the box.

It's also essential to have a thermos with a wide mouth (not the tall, beverage variety). The thermos makes packing leftovers and overnight crock pot soups a simple solution, especially at the end of the week when some of your other staples might be running low. Quick tip: Pour boiling water into your thermos while you are reheating the soup or leftovers, then pour out the water before filling. This will prime the thermos, keeping the food hot longer.

IN THE BOX

When you are packing your child's lunch, it's important to include all the nutrition they need, and also some of the foods they love. Otherwise, your carefully packed meal may end up in the cafeteria trash can. A well-rounded meal will include protein (meats, eggs, nuts, avocado, coconut), fiber (nuts, coconut, fruits, vegetables), and fresh fruits or vegetables. Finally, don't forget the water!

Always pack water, and not fruit juices. Kids don't need the sugar spike that the juice gives them, and water is the only thing that will truly hydrate them. If you want to give them a treat, you can pack flavor infused water, but don't add sweeteners like sugar or agave. If they have been Paleo for most of their lives, their taste buds won't crave really sweet things. If they are just starting out on the Paleo diet, their taste buds will acclimate quickly.

IF THEY PACK IT, THEY WILL EAT

The best way to get your kids to eat their healthy lunch is to let them pack it themselves. The sections of the bento box provide a great way to help them balance their meal. The biggest section can be used for a sandwich, chicken legs, or other kind of "main" course. The smaller sections are perfect for trail mix, cut fruits and veggies, and cookies or muffins.

It's your job to make sure there are plenty of healthy options on hand, and to give them the tools to make choices that are good for their bodies. Help them pack their lunches the first few times so they get the hang of it, and then they'll be able to do it on their own. They'll be proud of their independence, and they'll be more likely to eat their lunch!

BASIC FOOD LIST

Here is a food guideline to get you going. Remember, there is a little bit of wiggle room, as even the Paleo diet experts disagree about certain foods. If you are unsure, you should always do your own research and tailor your diet to your specific needs.

Vegetables and Sea Vegetables: You can eat any and all vegetables. In fact, you should eat a "rainbow" of vegetables, from red to violet, in order to give your body a wide variety of vitamins and nutrients. Sea veggies, like seaweed and algae, are especially good for you.

Fruits: Eat all the fruits. These can be fresh, cooked, or dried. However, if you're trying to lose weight or if you have a problem with tooth decay, you may want to limit dried fruits.

Meats, Fish & Eggs: You will eat a lot of meat and eggs on the Paleo diet, as did our hunter-gatherer ancestors. Protein plays a huge role in proper brain and muscle development, and since you're not going to eat any legumes or grains, meat and eggs become an even more important source of this vital building block.

It is always best to eat meat and eggs that came from pasture raised animals that were fed a diet similar to what they would eat in the wild. Always stay away from meats that have added preservatives or flavor enhancers, like nitrites or MSG. All different fish species are healthy choices, just be conscious of high mercury levels and choose fish with ecologically friendly harvesting practices. Here are some options: Turkey, chicken, goat, lamb, pork, organ meat (liver, gizzards, heart), game meats (pheasant, duck, deer, bison, goose, quail), beef, eggs (from chicken, duck, emu, etc), fish, shell fish, and fish eggs.

Nuts, Seeds, and Butters: All nuts and seeds are good, as well as the butters made from them. Keep in mind that peanuts are NOT nuts. They are legumes, and thus are NOT part of the Paleo diet. Almond butter makes a great replacement for peanut butter, and there are many mild nut butters that work well in baking.

Fats and Oils: Use fats and oils sparingly. Remember that you can not use grain oils, like corn oil or peanut oil. But there are a lot of great substitutes: lard, tallow, bacon grease, olive oil, coconut oil, walnut oil, avocado oil, hazelnut oil, flaxseed oil (unheated).

Drinks: Filtered or spring water should be your main drink. You can also add herbal tea, coconut water, and freshly juiced fruits and vegetables. Stay away from soda, bottled juice and juice drinks.

Seasoning: Most spices are fine, including sea salt (NOT refined iodized salt).

The following foods/beverages are okay in moderation, but you don't want to overdo them: Coffee, chocolate, caffeinated tea, raw honey, stevia, agave, grade B maple syrup.

Foods To Avoid

Cereal Grains: Wheat, rice, barley, corn millet, spelt, kamut, rice, amaranth, sorghum, rye, oats, quinoa, or anything made out of grains (flour, noodles, bread, crackers).

Legumes: All beans are out of the picture, including soybeans (tofu, too) and peanuts. Eliminate black beans, pintos, lentils, peas, lima beans, black-eyed peas, garbanzo beans (hummus), kidney beans, etc.

Sugar and Artificial Sweeteners: white sugar, brown sugar, turbinado sugar, refined maple syrup, high fructose corn syrup, corn syrup, molasses, refined honey, sucralose, aspartame, Splenda, Equal.

Highly Processed Oils and Most Vegetable Oils: Any oil that comes from a seed or legume is not acceptable, like soybean oil, corn oil, safflower oil, and grape seed oil. Also stay away from hydrogenated, partially hydrogenated and refined oils.

Dairy Products: This includes butter, yogurt, cheese and milk from cows, goats, sheep and buffalo. Basically, if it comes from an animal's teat, it is not allowed on the diet. However, that is up for debate in the Paleo community. Do your research. If you choose to eat some dairy, make sure that it is full-fat, raw (unpasteurized), organic and grass-fed, fermented dairy.

MAKE-AHEAD RECIPES

- Coconut-Cashew Bread -
- Amazing Flatbread -
- Peach Fruit Leathers -
- Kale Chips -
- Maple-Cinnamon Granola -
- Sweet Potato chips -
- Chicken Wings -
- All Day Applesauce -
- Chia Pudding -
- Spice Cookies -
- Apricot Squares -
- Trail Mix Granola Bars -

YIPPEE! IT'S LUNCHTIME!

Coconut-Cashew Bread

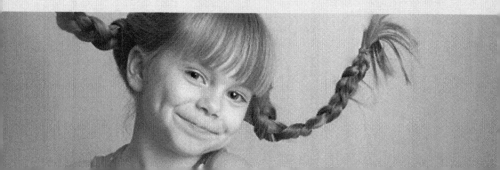

COCONUT-CASHEW BREAD

This dense, chewy bread stays together when you slice it and doesn't fall apart when you take a big bite of your sandwich. The psyllium seed fiber gives the dough elasticity. You can find psyllium husk powder in the stomach-aid sections of most health food stores. This recipe makes a small loaf, which can be sliced vertically for little finger sandwiches, or horizontally for larger "hoagie-style" ones.

Coconut-Cashew Bread Recipe

Ingredients:
- ¾ cup raw cashews
- 3 eggs, divided
- ¼ cup coconut milk
- ¼ cup coconut flour
- ¼ cup almond meal
- 4 tbsp melted coconut oil
- 1 tbsp psyllium husk powder (can be found in stomach-aid sections of most health food stores)
- 1 tsp cider vinegar
- 1 tsp sea salt
- 1 tsp baking soda

Directions:
Preheat oven to 350°F. Place cashews, egg yolks, vinegar, milk, and coconut oil into the canister of your food processor. Process until smooth.

To the cashew-egg mixture, add coconut flour, almond meal, psyllium husk powder and salt. Process until well incorporated.

In a medium sized bowl, beat egg whites with a wire whisk or electric mixer until stiff peaks form. Add the fluffy whites and the baking soda to the food processor and pulse several times until mixed.

Line the bottom and long sides of a 6" – 8" loaf pan with parchment paper. Lightly grease the short ends of the pan that are not covered with the paper. Spread the dough evenly in the pan.

Bake at 350°F for 45 – 55 minutes, until loaf is spongy and browned on the top. Increase time to 60 – 70 minutes for a double loaf baked in a larger pan. Allow to cool in the pan before removing. Store the bread in a paper bag for up to three days, or refrigerated up to a week.

Serving size: 1 slice   Yields: 6 servings

Prep time: 15 minutes   Bake time: 45 – 55 minutes   Total: 60 – 75 minutes

YIPPEE! IT'S LUNCHTIME!

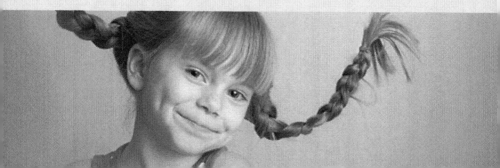

Amazing Flatbread

AMAZING FLATBREAD

The versatility of this recipe makes it a staple in our Paleo household. If you make your flatbread dough rounds large and thin, they can be used as tortillas or crepes. Made smaller with added oregano and basil, they are the perfect mini-pizza crust. Kids also love to make this bread because its short cooking time on the stovetop makes it an instant gratification recipe.

Amazing Flatbread Recipe

Ingredients:
- ½ cup coconut flour
- 2 tbsp psyllium husk powder (can be found in stomach-aid sections of most health food stores)
- ¼ cup coconut oil (or olive oil)
- 1 cup boiling water
- 1/8 tsp salt
- 1 tsp baking powder
- 1/8 tsp garlic powder (optional)

Directions:
Stir together flour, psyllium, salt, baking powder and garlic powder (if using). Add coconut oil in a scoop on top of flour mixture.

Slowly pour the boiling water over the coconut oil, mixing with a wooden spoon as the oil melts. You will end up with a nice ball of dough when finished. Heat a nonstick, cast iron skillet on a burner set to high heat. DO NOT put any oil in the skillet. Roll the dough into golf-ball sized rounds and flatten each round in the palms of your hands.

Place one round directly onto the hot skillet. Let it cook until the flatbread bubbles up a bit, and the skillet-side is starting to get brown, about two minutes. Flip and cook on the other side until dough is cooked through.

Repeat with each dough ball until all the dough is used. Store in a paper bag on the counter up to three days. This recipe can be refrigerated, but it might get a bit soft and spongy if kept in an airtight container.

Serving Size: 1 Round   Yields: 5 servings
Prep Time: 5 minutes   Cook Time: 15 – 20 minutes   Total: 20 – 25 minutes

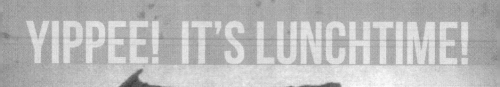

YIPPEE! IT'S LUNCHTIME!

YUM

Peach Fruit Leathers

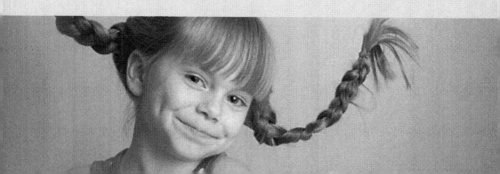

PEACH FRUIT LEATHERS

Unlike the popular prepackaged fruit-roll snacks, these homemade fruit leathers are 100% fruit with no added sugar, flavorings, or preservatives. Let your kids help wash the fruit, blend it, and pour it onto the parchment paper. When the leathers are all done and cooled, they can use a clean pair of scissors to cut them into all kinds of shapes to make their lunch box treat fun, delicious, and healthy!

Peach Fruit Leathers Recipe

Ingredients:
- 2 lbs fresh peaches

Directions:
Line the bottom of an 11" x 17" jelly roll pan with one large sheet of parchment paper. Set aside.

Wash the peaches. Slice them all the way around the center and twist to remove the pits. Cut peaches into chunks and place in the canister of your food processor.

Process until very smooth, at least five minutes or until the skins are reduced to tiny specs and all chunks of fruit are blended. (A high-powered processor, like a Vitamix, will be quicker.)

Pour processed fruit out onto the parchment paper and spread out even with a rubber spatula. Place the pan into the oven and turn the temperature to 170°F. Bake for 10 – 12 hours or until the peach puree is completely dehydrated with absolutely no soft, squishy spots.

Remove pan from oven and allow to cool. Once cooled, cut into rectangles (or shapes) with clean, dry scissors. Store in an airtight container or zipper bag up to two weeks.

Serving Size: One leather   Yields: 12 servings
Prep time: 15 minutes   Cook time: 10 – 12 hours   Total: 10 – 12 hrs, 15 minutes

YIPPEE! IT'S LUNCHTIME!

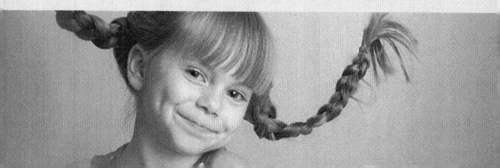

Kale Chips

KALE CHIPS

You will be surprised by how much your children will love to eat their greens with a bag of these healthy kale chips. They are easy to make and can take on nearly any kind of spice. Just keep in mind that it's best to use full-sized kale rather than the baby kale for this recipe, as the baby kale leaves become too delicate when baked.

Kale Chips Recipe

Ingredients:
- 1 bunch kale
- 1.5 tbsp olive oil
- 1 tsp salt, or spices to taste

Directions:
Preheat oven to 275°F.

Wash the kale and dry thoroughly either in a salad spinner, with a clean, fresh towel, or with paper towels. Trim off stems and tear the leaves into large pieces and place them in a bowl.

Toss the leaves with olive oil until completely coated, getting in there with your hands if necessary.

Line a cookie sheet with parchment paper. Spread the coated kale onto the parchment paper and bake at 275°F for thirty minutes, turning half way through bake time. Remove from oven when leaves are crisp, but not burned. Allow to cool on tray completely.

Sprinkle with salt or any other seasonings. Store in a sealed bag or container up to two weeks.

Serving Size: 1 Cup   Yields: about 4 servings
Prep time: 5 minutes   Bake time: 30 minutes   Total: 35 minutes

YIPPEE! IT'S LUNCHTIME!

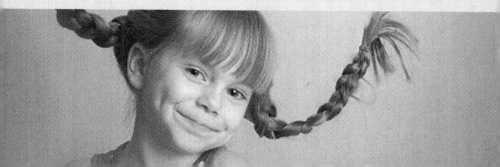

Maple-Cinnamon Granola

MAPLE-CINNAMON GRANOLA

Kids love cereal. It's crunchy and sweet. It's also quick, easy, and healthy... if it's made from nuts and seeds rather than grains and sugar! Whip up a batch of this delicious cinnamon granola to pair with almond milk for a crunchy good breakfast-for-lunch.

Maple-Cinnamon Granola Recipe

Ingredients:
- 1 cup raw almonds
- 1 cup raw cashews
- ½ cup flaked unsweetened coconut
- ¼ cup raw pumpkin seeds (shelled)
- ¼ cup raw sunflower seeds
- 1 tbsp hempseeds (optional)
- 1 tbsp flaxseeds
- 1/3 cup grade B maple syrup
- ¼ cup coconut oil
- ½ cup dried currants or raisins
- 1 tsp vanilla
- 1 tsp sea salt (optional)
- 1 tsp cinnamon
- ½ tsp nutmeg

Directions:
Preheat oven to 275°F. In a food processor, combine almonds, cashews, and coconut in the food processor. Pulse 5 – 8 times until chunked into small bits. Pour into a large glass bowl.

Combine coconut oil, vanilla, and maple syrup in a small saucepan. Melt over low heat, stirring constantly until completely melted.

To the nut mixture, add pumpkin seeds, sunflower seeds, flaxseeds, salt, cinnamon, and nutmeg. Stir to combine. Pour the coconut oil mixture over the top of the nuts and seeds and stir to coat.

Line an 11" x 17" jelly roll pan with parchment paper. Spread the granola mixture in an even layer across the lined pan. Bake at 275°F for 25 – 30 minutes until crunchy and golden. Remove from oven, sprinkle with currants or raisins, and press together with the back of a metal spatula to help chunks form. Allow to cool completely in pan.

Break into chunks and store in an airtight container up to two weeks.

Serving Size: 1 cup   Yields: 5 servings
Prep time: 15 minutes   Bake time: 30 minutes   Total: 45 minutes

YIPPEE! IT'S LUNCHTIME!

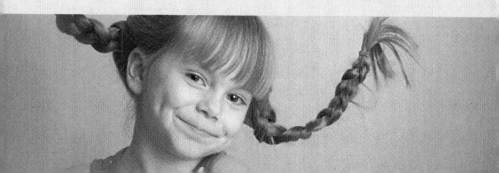

Sweet Potato Chips

SWEET POTATO CHIPS

Unfortunately, the sweet potato chips that have inundated the grocery stores are not quite fit for a Paleo diet because they are generally made with grain oils. But it's not so hard to make a batch of kettle-cooked, homemade sweet potato chips that will fulfill your child's appetite for a salty snack or crunchy side dish.

Sweet Potato Chip Recipe

Ingredients:
- 2-4 tablespoons olive oil or melted coconut oil (adjust to needs, potatoes need to be coated and glossy but not over-oily or they won't crisp up)
- 3 large sweet potatoes
- Sea salt to taste

Directions:
Preheat oven to 400 degrees and lightly grease 2 cookie sheets, or line with parchment paper.

Scrub or peel the sweet potatoes, removing any bad spots. Make sure to NOT rinse them, or the oil will not stick. Slice very thin with a sharp knife, or use a mandolin to get paper-thin slices.

Place sweet potatoes on the cookie sheet in a single layer, being careful not to crowd them or they will be too soft. If needed use two cookie sheets to ensure they have enough space and come out crispy. Coat with olive oil, or melted coconut oil and sprinkle sea salt on top. Place in the oven an bake for 8-10 minutes, then flip potatoes over and bake for another 5 minutes or until the edges go slightly brown and have curled up a bit. Allow to cool completely before storing in an airtight container. These will keep up to a few days, but probably won't last that long!

Serving Size: 1 cup   Yields: Varies, about five servings
Prep Time: 20 minutes   Cook time: 13-15 minutes   Total: 33-35 minutes

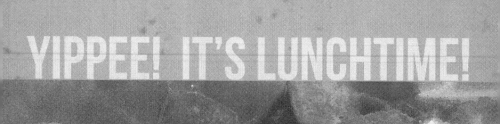

YIPPEE! IT'S LUNCHTIME!

Chicken Wings

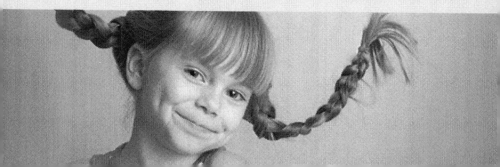

CHICKEN WINGS

Wildly popular with all the kids, chicken wings will make your child the envy of the lunch table. Pack them cold in the lunch box either plain with dips on the side, or toss them in this tasty teriyaki-inspired sauce.

Chicken Wings Recipe

Ingredients:
- 2 pounds chicken wings and legs, fresh or thawed

Sauce:
- 2 tbsp   liquid coconut aminos (can be found easily at health food stores in the Asian section)
- 1 tbsp   raw honey, melted
- 1 clove   garlic, crushed

Directions:
Preheat oven to 425° F. If the wings are coming out of the freezer, make sure they are thawed well and then dry them with a paper towel. Place wings on a cookie sheet. Bake for 30 minutes, then turn over for another 5 minutes or until crisp and golden.

To coat the wings with sauce: In a large bowl, whisk together all sauce ingredients. Place cooked wings into the sauce and toss to coat. Store in an airtight container in the refrigerator up to three days.

Serving Size: 5 wings   Yields: varies, about 5 servings
Prep time: 5 minutes   Cook time: 35 minutes   Total: 40 minutes

YIPPEE! IT'S LUNCHTIME!

All Day Applesauce

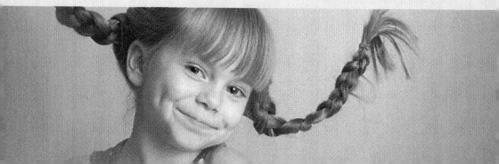

ALL DAY APPLESAUCE

Applesauce has always been one of my kids' favorites. While there are many options for 100% fruit prepackaged applesauce, nothing smells better than apples and cinnamon slow cooking all day in the crock-pot. You can give the applesauce responsibility completely to even your youngest child, and they will be so proud of what they've made for the family.

All Day Applesauce Recipe

Ingredients:
- 3 lbs fresh apples, any variety
- 1 tsp cinnamon (optional)
- ½ cup filtered water

Directions:
Peel and core the apples. Cut into large chunks and place in the bowl of a medium sized slow cooker. Sprinkle apples with cinnamon and water. Cook in the slow cooker 6 hours for light, chunky sauce and up to eight hours for dark, smooth sauce. Stir with a spoon to smooth together any chunks. Remove to an airtight container and refrigerate up to five days.

*Cook the apples for 12+ hours for apple butter.

Serving size: ½ cup   Yields: 4 – 6 servings
Prep time: 15 minutes   Cook time: 6 – 8 hours   Total: 6 – 8 hr, 15 minutes

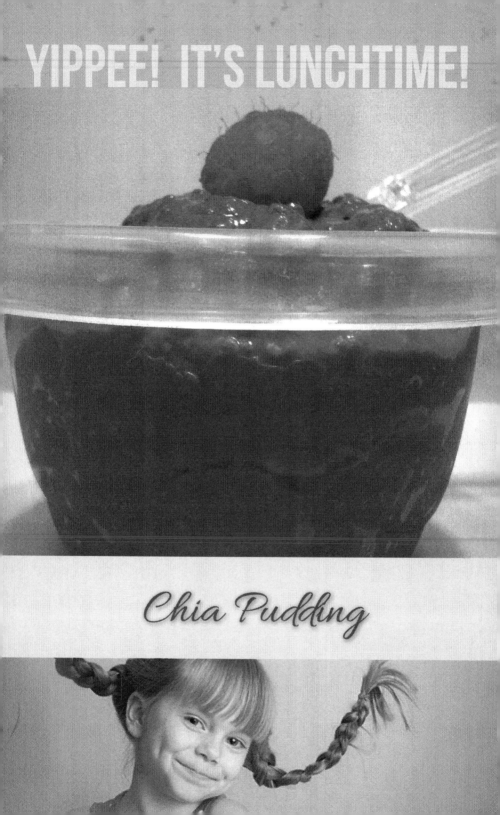

YIPPEE! IT'S LUNCHTIME!

Chia Pudding

CHIA PUDDING

There are a number of ways to make pudding "snack-packs" that don't include processed sugars and artificial coloring. This recipe uses chia seeds to turn the coconut milk from a creamy liquid to the fluffy, chocolate mousse style pudding. Chia seeds are full of nutrients and are rich in Omega-3 fatty acids, so this little pudding cup packs a huge health punch!

Chia Pudding Recipe

Ingredients:
- 1 14oz can full-fat coconut milk
- 2/3 cup white chia seeds
- 3 tbsp raw cocoa powder (or 1 tbsp vanilla for vanilla pudding)
- 2 tbsp xylitol or melted raw honey

Directions:
Place all ingredients in a container with a tight-fitting lid. Shake until everything is mixed well. Pour into individual containers with lids, or one large lidded container. Refrigerate overnight.

This pudding will retain a slight crunch from the seeds, which do not turn completely soft. If your child doesn't love the crunch, sprinkle the pudding with granola, raspberries, or toasted coconut to disguise the crunch inside!

Serving size: ½ cup   Yields: 6 servings
Prep time: 5 minutes   Refrigeration time: over night

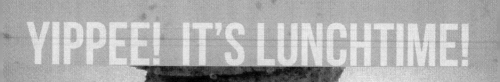

YIPPEE! IT'S LUNCHTIME!

Spice Cookies

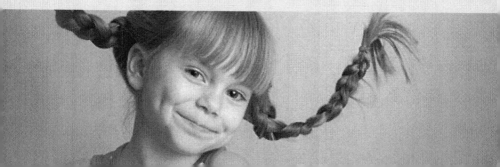

SPICE COOKIES

Even the pickiest eaters devour this healthy alternative to the sugar cutout cookie. Let the older children do the mixing and the youngest can cut shapes with their favorite cookie cutters and decorate the unbaked cookies with seeds, nuts, and dried fruit. This is a very special, and much appreciated lunch-box treat!

Spice Cookie Recipe

Ingredients:
- 2 cups almond meal
- 3 tbsp grass-fed butter or coconut oil
- 3 tbsp pure maple syrup
- ½ tsp baking soda
- ½ tsp cinnamon, plus some for sprinkling
- ½ tsp nutmeg
- 1 tsp xylitol (for sprinkling- optional)

Directions:
In a large bowl, mix almond meal, cinnamon, nutmeg, and baking soda with a wooden spoon. Mix in maple syrup and butter or coconut oil until batter is smooth. Wrap tightly in wax paper and refrigerate one hour.

Preheat oven to 325°F. Remove dough from refrigerator and set between two sheets of wax or parchment paper. Roll to ¼ inch thickness.

Cut into shapes with cookies cutters and place cut dough onto a parchment-lined cookie sheet. Decorate with nuts and dried fruits or dust with cinnamon, if desired. Bake 8 – 10 minutes until cookies are set through and starting to brown on top. Remove from oven, sprinkle with xylitol (optional) and cool on the cookie sheet.

Store in an airtight container up to one week.

Serving Size: 3 small cookies   Yields: 6 servings
Prep time: 10 minutes + 1 hour refrigeration (dough)
Prep for baking: 10 minutes, rolling and cutting
Bake time: 8 – 10 minutes   Total time: 1 hour, 30 minutes

YIPPEE! IT'S LUNCHTIME!

Apricot Bars

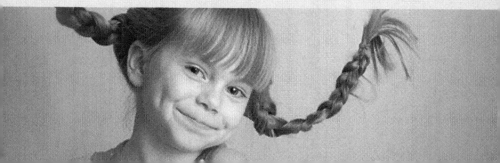

APRICOT BARS

These delicious dessert bars are the perfect blend of sweet and tart without any added sugars. The apricot bars taste good right out of the freezer, but you can pack them frozen in the lunch box and they will keep their shape while keeping the rest of the food cool!

Apricot Bar Recipe

Ingredients:
- 2 cups unsulphured dried apricots
- 1 cup white raisins
- 1 ¼ cup raw pecans
- ¾ cup shredded, unsweetened coconut
- 2 tbsp coconut oil
- ½ tsp vanilla

Directions:
Place apricots, raisins, 1-cup pecans, ½ cup coconut, 1 ½ tbsp coconut oil, and vanilla into the bowl of your food processor. Pulse until the mixture forms a mealy dough.

Grease the bottom and sides of an 8" x 8" glass baking dish with the remaining coconut oil.

Pour the mixture into the pan and press with your clean hands until the bars are flattened and filling in all the corners. Sprinkle with remaining coconut and pecans (chopped). Cover with a tight-fitting lid or wrap and freeze until firm. Cut into squares.

Serving size: 1 square   Yields: 12 squares
Prep time: 10 minutes   Freeze time: 1 hour or more

YIPPEE! IT'S LUNCHTIME!

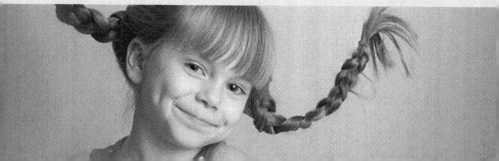

Trail Mix Granola Bars

TRAIL MIX GRANOLA BARS

This granola bar recipe is simple to throw together and free of almost all common allergens and can be made vegan, so it's a good one to make for a play date or when it's your turn to bring the snack for soccer practice. You can adapt the flavors by using your favorite add-ins, like dried cherries and raw cocoa nibs, or dried apples and cinnamon.

Trail Mix Granola Bar Recipe

Ingredients:
- 1 cup shredded coconut
- ½ cup almond meal
- ½ cup pepitas (shelled pumpkin seeds)
- ½ cup slivered almonds
- ½ cup sunflower seeds
- ¼ cup almond butter
- ¼ cup raw honey (or maple syrup)
- 2 tbsp coconut oil
- 1 tbsp flax seeds
- 1 tbsp flax meal
- 1 ½ tbsp water
- 1 tsp vanilla
- ½ cup add-ins, like dried fruits or cocoa nibs (I used currants)
- Pinch sea salt (optional)

Directions:
Preheat oven to 325°F.

In a large bowl, mix together flax meal and water and let rest for three minutes. Add in the coconut oil, raw honey, almond butter, and vanilla. Mix with a wooden spoon until smooth.

Add remaining ingredients and mix until evenly incorporated.
Oil an 8" x 8" metal baking pan with coconut oil. Pour in the granola bar mixture and press into the corners with a rubber spatula. Press the top down and smooth it out.

Bake on the middle rack for 22 – 25 minutes until the edges and top are golden brown and center is set. Cool in pan completely before cutting into twelve bars. Store in an airtight container for up to one week.

Serving size: 1 bar   Yields: 12 servings
Prep time: 7 minutes   Bake time: 22 – 25 minutes   Total: 30 minutes

QUICK-PACK RECIPES

- Almond Butter and Banana Sandwich -
- Egg Salad Sandwich -
- Simple Salad -
- Turkey Club Sandwich -
- Ants Off The Log -
- Mexican Beef Lettuce Wraps with Mango Salsa -
- Dilled Cucumbers -
- Chinese Chicken Lettuce Wraps -
- Sausage-N-Apple Spears -
- Before-School Chili -
- Taco Seasoning -
- Savory Poppers -

YIPPEE! IT'S LUNCHTIME!

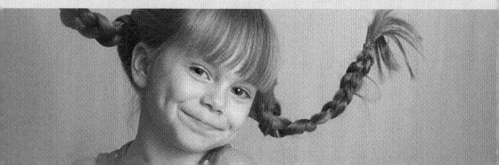

Almond Butter & Banana Sandwich

ALMOND BUTTER AND BANANA SANDWICH

This sandwich is one of our household favorites. If you keep the coconut-cashew bread on hand, it will make packing lunch a cinch.

Almond Butter And Banana Sandwich Recipe

Ingredients:
- 2 five-inch slices of coconut-cashew bread
- 1 tbsp almond butter
- 1 tsp raw honey
- ½ cup sliced bananas

Directions:
Spread the almond butter on one slice of bread. Spread the raw honey on the other slice of bread. Slice the banana and place it evenly across the almond butter. Put the honeyed bread on top of the almond butter and banana bread slice.

Serving size: 1 sandwich   Yields: 1 serving
Prep time: 5 minutes

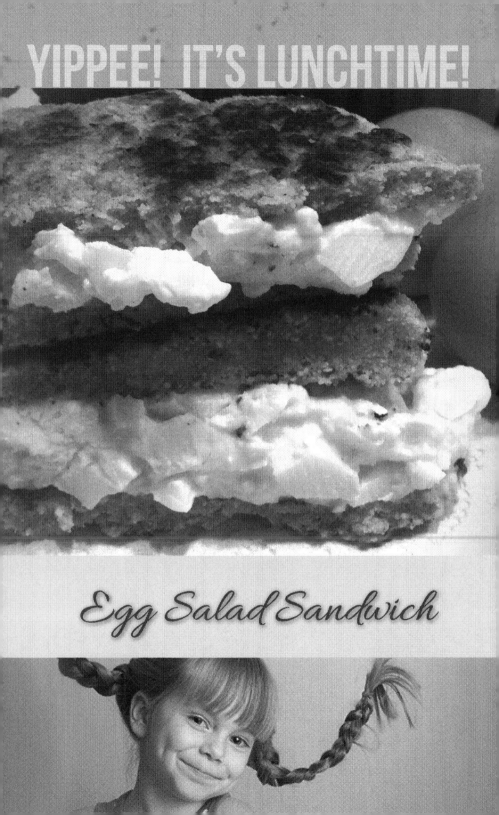

YIPPEE! IT'S LUNCHTIME!

Egg Salad Sandwich

EGG SALAD SANDWICH

If you keep boiled eggs in the refrigerator, this recipe is a snap. You can serve it between two pieces of flatbread or in a simple, fresh lettuce wrap. Pair with kale chips and a piece of fruit and you have a well-balanced, delicious lunch for kids of any age.

Egg Salad Sandwich Recipe

Ingredients:
- 2 boiled eggs
- 1 tbsp Paleo mayonnaise
- Salt and pepper to taste

Directions:
Peel the eggs and place in a small bowl. Break them up with the back of a fork. Add the mayonnaise, salt and pepper. Mix and mash with the fork until the egg salad is mixed well but still chunky. Spread between two pieces of flatbread, or serve with lettuce wraps.

Serving size: 1 sandwich   Yields: 1 serving
Prep time: 5 minutes

YIPPEE! IT'S LUNCHTIME!

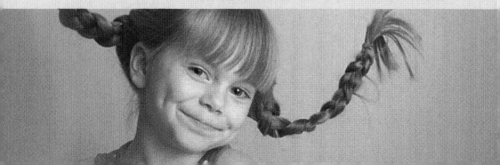

Simple Salad
& Lemon Poppy Seed Dressing

SIMPLE SALAD WITH LEMON POPPY SEED DRESSING

A simple salad has to be one of the easiest Paleo recipes of all time. If you are sticking to a strict Paleo diet, you should already have a fridge full of fruits, veggies, and meats ripe for the picking. Mix and match your child's favorites, or use this recipe as a guideline. Sprinkle the salad with a handful of seeds, and you have a well-rounded meal all in one container. This is especially good for the teen's lunch box (or your own).

Simple Salad Recipe

Ingredients:
- 2 cups lettuce (romaine, red leaf, iceberg, or other)
- Small Roma tomato
- ½ cup cubed, cooked chicken
- ¼ cup diced cucumber
- ¼ cup shredded carrot
- Any other toppings (sunflower seeds, almonds, boiled egg, raisins, apples, bacon bits, etc.)

Lemon Poppy Seed Dressing

Ingredients:
- 1 tbsp   extra virgin olive oil
- 1 tbsp lemon juice
- ¼ tsp poppy seeds
- 1/8 tsp ground mustard (optional)
- Pinch of salt and pepper

Directions:
For the salad: Wash and dry the lettuce and tear it into bite sized pieces. Place lettuce in a lidded container. Wash and dice the tomato and add it to the lettuce. Cube the chicken (leftover roasted or grilled chicken works great), and add it to the salad. Peel and dice the cucumber and add it as well. Peel the outer layer off of a carrot, and then use the peeler to peel down the rest of the carrot. Add the peels/shreds to the salad.

For the dressing: Place all ingredients in a small container and put the lid on tightly. Shake until well mixed. You will have to shake again before pouring on the salad.

Serve with a couple slices of coconut-cashew or almond bread spread with grass-fed butter or pesto.

Serving size: 1 salad   Yields: 1 serving
Prep time: 10 minutes

YIPPEE! IT'S LUNCHTIME!

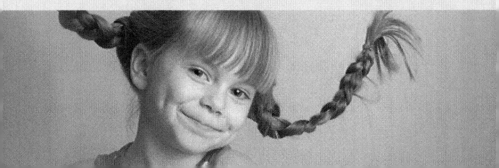

Turkey Club Sandwich

TURKEY CLUB SANDWICH

My son told me this was the best sandwich he had ever eaten. This is a great deli-style sandwich for older kids and those with bigger appetites. If you keep the bread on hand, it's a quick sandwich fix. If not, you can always roll the ingredients in a large leaf of crisp iceberg lettuce or kale.

Turkey Club Sandwich Recipe

Ingredients:
- 2 large slices of coconut-cashew bread (cut lengthwise, hoagie style)
- 2 thick cut slices of natural deli-cut roasted turkey breast
- 2 slices precooked bacon (maybe leftover from yesterday's breakfast)
- 2 slices tomato
- 1 -2 leaves lettuce (any variety), washed and dried
- 1 tbsp Paleo mayonnaise

Directions:
Spread the mayonnaise on one piece of bread. Top with turkey breast, tomato, bacon, and lettuce. Make sure the lettuce is on top of the tomato to prevent the juices from soaking into the bread. Pack with sweet potato chips and applesauce for a well-rounded, hearty lunch.

Serving size: 1 sandwich   Yields: 1 serving
Prep time: 5 minutes

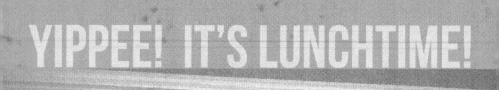

YIPPEE! IT'S LUNCHTIME!

Ants Off The Log

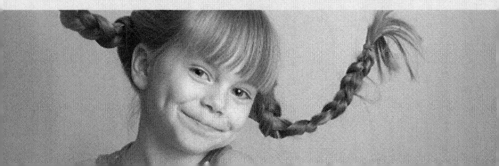

ANTS OFF THE LOG

Ants-on-a-log are those wonderful childhood snacks made from celery stick logs and raisin ants stuck down with peanut butter. Well, try as I might, almond butter just doesn't stick the ants to the log. Because it doesn't have any added sugar, almond butter is generally a bit runny. While that's not good for sticking power, it's excellent for dipping! Smaller children love this simple lunch, and older kids enjoy it for lunch or an after-school snack! Moms love it because it's easy and healthy.

Ants Off The Log Recipe

Ingredients:
- ½ cup almond butter
- Large carrot, peeled and sliced into sticks
- Large celery stalk, washed, trimmed, and cut into sticks
- ¼ cup raisins or currants

Directions:
Place the washed, cut vegetables into one compartment of a bento box. Pour the almond butter into a small compartment of the bento box and top with currants or raisins. Your child can dip in their "logs" and save the "ants" from drowning in a sticky pool of goodness! Add a trail mix granola bar or a piece of fruit and your lunch box is complete!

Serving size: 1 bento lunch   Yields: 1 serving
Prep time: 5 minutes

YIPPEE! IT'S LUNCHTIME!

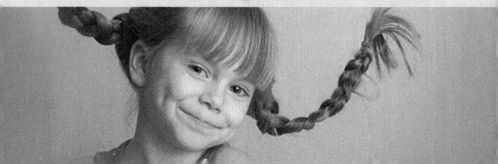

Mexican Beef Lettuce Wraps & Mango Salsa

MEXICAN BEEF LETTUCE WRAPS WITH MANGO SALSA

Unlike the "walking taco" that has become so popular among the school-lunch fare, this portable Mexican lunch is good for growing bodies! Oh... in case you didn't know, the "walking taco" is seasoned beef, sour cream, and cheese sauce poured into an open bag of corn chips.

Mexican Beef Lettuce Wraps Recipe

Ingredients:
- ¼ lb thin-sliced roast beef, from leftover roast or from the deli counter (grass fed, organic- as always)
- ½ tsp taco seasoning (see recipe pg.59)
- 4 – 5 iceberg lettuce cups
- 1 serving quick mango salsa (recipe follows)

Directions:
In a small bowl, toss the slices of roast beef in the taco seasoning to coat, adding salt and pepper to taste. Place in one compartment of your bento box.

To make lettuce cups: Peel the outer layers off of one fresh head of iceberg lettuce. Turn the head on its side. With a large knife, cut off the "top" of the head about 4 inched down. This should make at least a dozen "cups" in various sizes. Wash and dry them before placing 4 – 5 in a section of the bento box. Store the rest wrapped in paper towel or clean towel in a bag or food storage bin in the refrigerator.

Quick Mango Salsa Directions:
Peel the skin off on one fresh mango. Using a sharp paring knife, cut the flesh away from the pit. Discard pit. Dice flesh into ¼ inch pieces and place in a small bowl.

Wash one small Roma tomato. Slice down the middle and discard seeds. Dice into ¼ inch pieces and add to mango.

Wash and finely chop one small bunch of cilantro. Add one tablespoon of the chopped cilantro to the mango. Add one small clove garlic, crushed and ½ teaspoon fresh chopped jalapeno pepper (seeds removed). Chop one green onion (white and pale green parts only) and add it.

Squeeze the juice of ¼ lime over the top of the mango mixture. Salt and pepper to taste and toss everything together to coat completely. Pour salsa into one small section of the bento box.

Make sure to pack a spoon and fork for building the lettuce cups... and napkins, because this might get juicy!

Serving size: 1 bento lunch   Yields: 1 serving
Prep time: 15 minutes

YIPPEE! IT'S LUNCHTIME!

Dilled Cucumbers

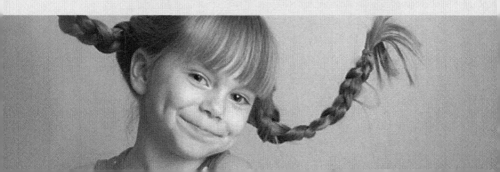

DILLED CUCUMBERS

My daughter adores pickles, but just try to find a jar of pickles at the local grocery store that doesn't have food dye and a lot of salt. We try to make our own pickles, but when our stockpile of cucumber-dill filled mason jars runs out, this simple recipe will suffice. It's fresh, crunchy, with just enough flavor kick to take a serving of veggies (well, cukes are actually fruits) up a notch!

Dilled Cucumber Recipe

Ingredients:
- 1 cup cucumbers, washed and sliced (I used baby cukes sliced vertically, but full-sized cucumber sliced into rounds or spears also works well)
- 1 tsp apple cider vinegar
- ¼ tsp dried dill (or ½ tsp fresh, chopped dill)
- Healthy pinch of sea salt

Directions:
Toss all ingredients together in a small bowl or zip-top bag until completely coated. Pack right away or store in refrigerator up to three days. These are especially good served with the egg salad pita sandwich!

Serving Size: 5 – 6 baby dilled cucumbers   Yields: 1 serving
Prep time: 5 minutes

YIPPEE! IT'S LUNCHTIME!

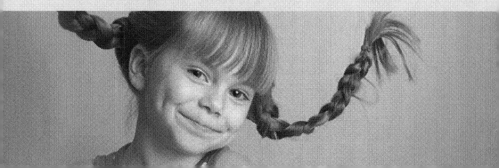

Chinese Chicken Lettuce Wraps

CHINESE CHICKEN LETTUCE WRAPS

These lettuce wraps are full of delicious flavors and textures, just like the wraps from the mainstream Chinese restaurants. In a pinch, you can substitute different seeds for the pepitos and even pork in place of chicken. The recipe is versatile and easy to toss together on a busy school day morning.

Chinese Chicken Lettuce Wrap Recipe

Ingredients:
- ½ cup cooked chicken (grilled or roasted- leftover is great)
- ¼ cup shredded carrots
- 1 tbsp chopped green onion
- 1 tbsp pepitas or slivered almonds
- 1 clove garlic, crushed
- 1 tbsp liquid coconut aminos (can be found easily at health food stores in the Asian section)
- 1 tsp raw honey (optional)
- ½ tsp lemon juice
- ¼ tsp red pepper flakes (optional)
- 4 – 5 iceberg lettuce cups

Directions:
Cut the chicken into ½ inch cubes or chunks and set in a medium bowl with the shredded carrots, chopped green onion, and pepitas.

In a small bowl, whisk together the coconut aminos, raw honey, lemon juice, red pepper flakes and garlic. Pour the sauce over the chicken mixture and toss to coat.

Serve in a bento box with four to five lettuce cups. Don't forget the utensils!

Serving Size: 4 – 5 lettuce filled lettuce cups   Yields: 1 serving
Prep time: 10 minutes

YIPPEE! IT'S LUNCHTIME!

Sausage-N-Apple Spears

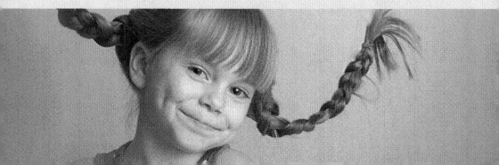

SAUSAGE-N-APPLE SPEARS

Kids love to eat things off of sticks. No, really, it's a fact. Just remember that if you are packing this sausage kebab for younger children, you'll want to cut the tip off the end of the skewer after you've loaded it up... just so no-one gets hurt!

Sausage-N-Apple Spears Recipe

Ingredients:
- Small Gala apple
- Cooked sausage, any variety
- 1 tsp lemon juice
- 1 tbsp cashew butter, for dipping
- Skewers

Directions:
Wash and core the apple. Cut into one-inch chunks. Place apple chunks in a small bowl and toss with the lemon juice to prevent the apples from browning. Cut sausage into 6 – 8 rounds. Slide the apples and sausages onto the skewer by inserting the pointed end into the center of each piece and sliding it back toward the center of the skewer. Alternate apples and sausage until everything has been used.

Remember to gauge your skewer size to your lunch box size. You can always snip the ends of the skewers down to fit before you fill them with meats and fruits.

Serve with cashew butter for dipping and a side of crunchy kale chips!

Serving Size: 2 – 3 fully loaded skewers   Yields: 1 serving
Prep time: 7 minutes

YIPPEE! IT'S LUNCHTIME!

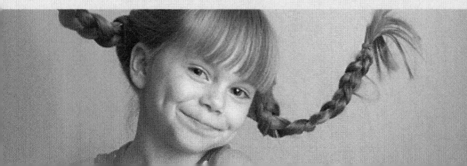

Before School Chili

BEFORE SCHOOL CHILI

Chili is such a filling, flavorful comfort food that my family eats it at least once a week. The problem is that there are rarely leftovers because we don't have a pot big enough to hold a batch that will yield enough to save. While we work on remedying that situation, I have found a way to get a quick chili fix in about fifteen minutes so we have chili on demand! It goes straight from the pot to the thermos in the morning and I know my kids will have full bellies at lunchtime.

Before School Chili Recipe

Ingredients:
- 1 lb lean ground beef
- Medium white onion
- Bell pepper (green, red, or yellow)
- 1 quart home-canned diced tomatoes (or 28 oz can store-bought)
- 2 tbsp taco seasoning (see recipe pg.59)
- Salt and pepper to taste

Directions:
Wash the bell pepper, then slice it in half and remove the seeds and stem. Dice the pepper and set aside.

Peel the outer layer off of the onion. Remove the top and base and chop the remaining onion.

Place the ground beef, onion, and bell pepper in a medium heavy pot on the stovetop set over medium-high heat. Stir regularly until the meat is browned and the onion is translucent, about ten minutes.

Add the tomatoes, taco seasoning, salt and pepper. Stir and heat until the chili is heated through. Pour about one cup of chili into a clean, warm thermos and screw the lid tight!

Serving size: about 1 cup   Yields: 5 servings
Prep time: 5 minutes   Cook time: 10 minutes   Total: 15 minutes

YIPPEE! IT'S LUNCHTIME!

Taco Seasoning

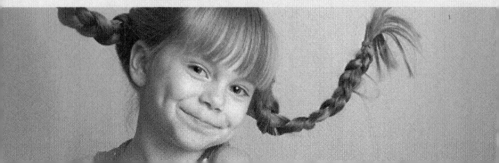

TACO SEASONING

This is a seasoning I keep on hand at all times. You can toss it with just about any meat for a quick lettuce wrap filling, add it to soups or burgers, and of course, make fast chili!

Taco Seasoning Recipe

Ingredients:
- 2 tbsp chili powder
- 4 tsp ground cumin
- 1 tsp garlic powder
- 1 tsp smoked paprika
- ½ tsp onion powder
- ½ tsp crushed red pepper flakes
- ½ tsp dried oregano
- Sea salt and ground black pepper to taste

Directions:
Mix all ingredients together and store in a glass spice jar with a tight-fitting lid. This spice blend will keep for at least a month, but likely won't last that long!

Serving Size: 1 small glass spice jar
Yields: several servings depending on amount used
Prep time: 5 minutes

YIPPEE! IT'S LUNCHTIME!

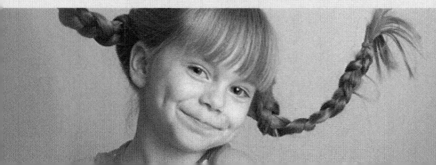

Savory Poppers

SAVORY POPPERS

This incredible batter is so simple, it's almost unbelievable. With just a couple of ingredients, you have a delicious and fluffy base for savory muffins, pancakes, or quick flatbread rounds. In this recipe, I'll use the batter in mini-muffin tins and stuff it with a hearty filling for a quick lunch box meal.

Remember, if you don't include the ingredients I'm using in your version of the Paleo diet, like grass-fed cheese, please feel free to substitute another filling. Bacon and chives are also delicious in this one!

Savory Poppers Recipe

Ingredients:
- 2 large eggs
- ¼ cup full-fat coconut milk
- ¼ cup coconut flour
- ½ tsp baking powder
- Pinch sea salt
- Coconut oil or grass-fed butter for pan

Filling:
- ¼ cup uncured smoked ham, diced
- ¼ cup grass-fed cheese, crumbled

Directions:
Preheat oven to 450°F. Grease 9 cups of a mini-muffin pan with oil.
In a medium bowl, whisk together the eggs and coconut milk. In a separate bowl, mix together coconut flour, baking powder and sea salt. Stir flour mixture into egg mixture. The batter will resemble thick pancake batter.

Scoop one tablespoon of batter into each of the nine oiled muffin cups. Mix together the ham and cheese (or other filling). Take one pinch of filling and gently push it down into one uncooked muffin at a time, allowing some of the batter to come over the top.

Bake for about ten minutes until the poppers are fluffy and golden brown on top. Remove poppers from the tin right away and allow to cool on a wire rack. Pack in a wax bag or bento box with a side of applesauce and an almond cookie or two.

These poppers will stay in the refrigerator up to three days, and can be frozen but might deflate a bit in the freezer.

*This batter can also be fried in a hot, oiled skillet and used like a pancake or a quick sandwich round. Fry for about two minutes over medium-high heat on one side, flip, and continue frying for about one minute on the other side until the edges are crispy and the dough is cooked through.

Serving size: 3 poppers   Yields: 3 servings   Prep time: 7 minutes
Bake time: 10 minutes   Total: 17 minutes

BEVERAGES

- Pineapple Mint Water -
- Strawberry Grape Water -
- Strawberry Milk -

YIPPEE! IT'S LUNCHTIME!

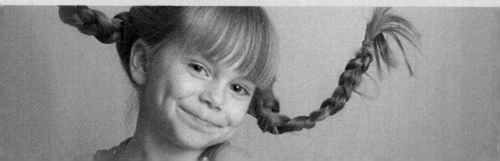

Pineapple Mint Water

PINEAPPLE MINT WATER

It is so important for kids to stay hydrated throughout the day. Dehydration can cause headaches, stomachaches, fatigue, and lead to a number of other health and behavioral problems. But kids don't always just want plain water. This flavor-infused water is just as good for your kids, but adds a little sweetness... naturally. In fact, the mint in this drink can aid digestion and calm an upset stomach.

Pineapple Mint Water Recipe

Ingredients:
- 5 chunks fresh or frozen pineapple
- 5 fresh mint leaves
- Filtered water to fill pint jar

Directions:
Place the pineapple and mint in the bottom of a clean pint jar. Add water (or water and ice) to fill the jar to the rim. Screw on the lid and refrigerate overnight.

To pack in the lunch, pour the water through a fine sieve into a water bottle or thermos. Older kids might want to drink it straight from the jar, or you can make this in a BPA-free plastic wide-mouthed water bottle and skip the jar entirely.

Serving size: 1 pint   Yields: 1 serving
Prep time: 5 minutes   Cool time: over night

YIPPEE! IT'S LUNCHTIME!

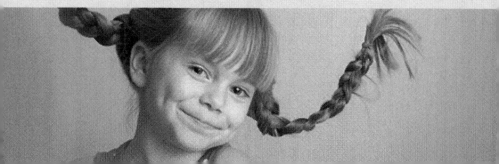

Strawberry Grape Water

STRAWBERRY GRAPE WATER

Another take on the flavored water infusion, this blend of strawberries and purple grapes adds a touch of fruit-punch taste to the water. If you want to make it a bit sweet, add some mottled fresh stevia leaves to the mix before cooling.

Strawberry Grape Water Recipe

Ingredients:
- Large strawberries
- 6 purple grapes
- Water to fill a pint jar

Directions:
Wash the strawberries and remove stems. Slice them in half or quarters. Wash the grapes and slice in half. Put all the fruit and slightly mottled stevia leaves, if desired, in a clean pint jar. Fill the rest of the jar to the rim with cold water and ice (optional). Screw on the lid and refrigerate overnight.

To pack, pour the water through a fine sieve into a water bottle or thermos. Older kids may want to drink straight from the jar, or you can use BPA-free plastic wide-mouth water bottles to make the flavor-water and skip the glass jar entirely.

Serving size: 1 pint   Yields: 1 serving
Prep time: 5 minutes   Cool time: over night

YIPPEE! IT'S LUNCHTIME!

Strawberry Milk

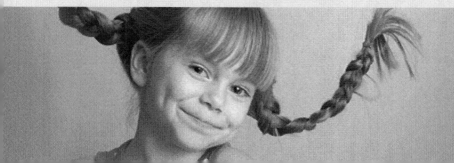

STRAWBERRY MILK

While I'm not an advocate of sugary drinks, I do believe that a treat once in a while is okay. My kids really enjoy a glass of milk with their spice cookies or their almond butter sandwiches, and this naturally pink strawberry milk is a fun way to add flair to their lunch box or afternoon snack. I used strawberries, but you could try it with raspberries or blackberries as well!

Strawberry Milk Recipe

Ingredients:
- 1 cup whole, fresh strawberries
- 1 cup plain almond milk
- ½ tsp raw honey

Directions:
Wash the strawberries and remove stems. Place berries in a bowl and smash with the back of a fork until you end up with a juicy, chunky sauce.

Pour the strawberry sauce, almond milk, and raw honey in a mason jar with a tight-fitting lid. Shake until everything is well blended, about a minute. At this point, you can leave the milk in the refrigerator overnight to achieve maximum flavor, or you can skip straight to straining.

To serve: Pour the milk through a fine mesh strainer into a lidded cup, thermos, or bottle. As you pour, mash down the pulp with the back of a spoon to make sure you are getting all of the delicious juices.

Serving size: 1 ¼ cup   Yields: 1 serving
Prep time: 5 minutes   Refrigeration time: overnight (optional)

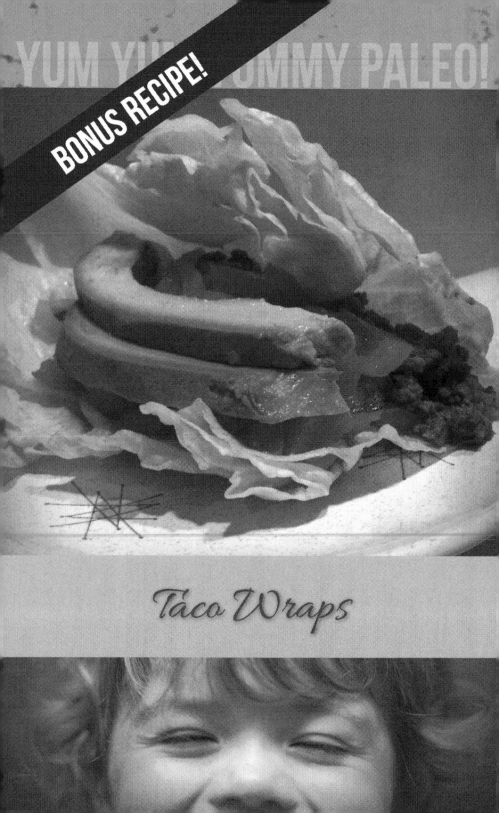

BONUS RECIPE!

YUM YUM YUMMY PALEO!

Taco Wraps

TACO WRAPS
(BONUS RECIPE FROM *THE PALEO KID*)

Taco night is a family tradition stemming from my own childhood. Every Friday night my dad would season and cook the meat while my brother and I chopped vegetables and set the table. My own kids love this tradition. We put all the ingredients on a large serving platter on a lazy susan in the middle of the table, and we assemble our own tacos as we chat and laugh and eat!

Taco Wrap Recipe

Ingredients:
- 1 lb ground beef
- 1 head iceberg lettuce
- 1 tomato
- 2 peppers (yellow, green, red- choose two)
- 1 small onion
- 1 tsp cumin
- 1 tsp garlic powder
- 1 tsp chili powder (or smoked paprika)
- 1 tbsp olive oil
- Salt and pepper to taste
- 1 avocado, sliced (for topping)
- Cilantro (garnish)

Directions:
Dice the vegetables (except avocado). In a large pan over medium heat, brown ground beef with spices, about 8 minutes. In another pan, heat olive oil over medium-high heat. Toss in vegetables and saute until just cooked, about five minutes. Slice avocado and dice tomato.

Rinse head of lettuce, peeling away any flimsy outside layers. Cut horizontally down the center. Use the "top" slices as cups for your taco wraps.
Pile the lettuce cups with meat and vegetables. Top with avocado slices and fresh cilantro. Fold over and enjoy!

Serving Size: 2 taco wraps   Yields: 5 servings   Prep Time: 10 minutes
Cook Time: 13 – 15 minutes   Total: 25 minutes

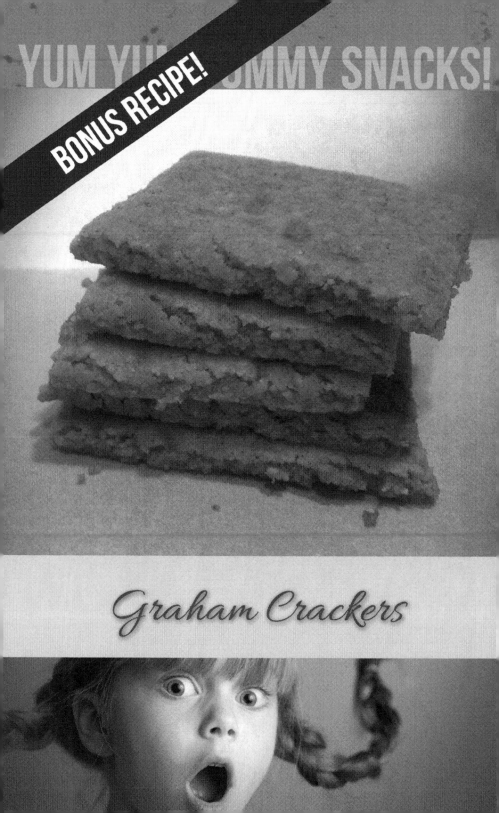

YUM YUM YUMMY SNACKS!

BONUS RECIPE!

Graham Crackers

GRAHAM CRACKERS
(BONUS RECIPE FROM *PALEO KID SNACKS*)

I recently took these crackers to a play date, and just about every parent there asked me for the recipe! I had one mom tell me that she couldn't stop eating them. Make a double batch of almond graham crackers and keep them in a sealed container. I'd say that they'll keep up to a week, but they probably won't last until tomorrow!

Graham Crackers Recipe

Ingredients:

- 2 ¼ c.   Blanched almond meal (or finely ground almonds)
- 3 tbsp   Coconut oil
- 3 tbsp   Grade B maple syrup
- 1 tsp   Cinnamon
- 1 tsp   Vanilla extract
- ¼ tsp   Baking soda

Directions:

Preheat oven to 325°F. Line a baking sheet with parchment paper.

Place all ingredients into a medium sized bowl. Mix with a hand mixer set on low until all ingredients are well blended and a dough ball begins to form. Remove the dough ball to the parchment-lined baking sheet.

Cover the dough ball with another sheet of parchment. With a rolling pin, roll out the dough until it is very thin, about 1/8 inch. Discard the top sheet of parchment. Prick the dough with a fork every few inches.

Bake in a preheated oven for 12 – 15 minutes, until the crackers are browned and firm to the touch. Remove from oven and cut immediately into 2-inch squares with a pizza cutter or large, sharp knife. Allow to cool in pan.

When the crackers are cooled, serve plain or topped with a dollop of apple butter! Store in an airtight container for up to 10 days.

Serving size: 3 crackers   Yields: 8 servings (24 crackers)
Prep time: 15 minutes   Cook time: 15 minutes
Total time: 30 minutes

ABOUT THE AUTHOR

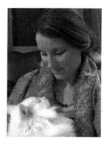

Kate Evans Scott is a stay-at-home mom to a preschooler and a toddler. In her former life she worked in graphic design and publishing which she now draws from to create inspiring books for young children and parents.

Her passion for writing began with her preschooler who is an encyclopedia of all things animal, vegetable and mineral. With a deep interest to create books that satisfy his desire to learn, and his love of food, Kids Love Press was born.

MORE BOOKS FROM KIDS LOVE PRESS:

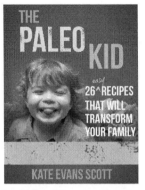

Available Now on Amazon

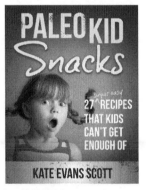

Available Now on Amazon

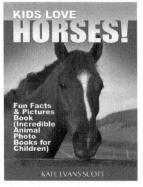

Available Now on Amazon

NOTES

NOTES

NOTES

43272050R00050

Made in the USA
Middletown, DE
05 May 2017